The Secret

To

A Healthy Digestion

How Warm And Cold Foods Affect Your Health

By Tansy Briggs, DOM

Integrative Oriental Medicine Practitioner

Copyright 2015

Tansy Briggs

Contents

Introduction

How are you supposed to know what's truly good for your body when a new fad diet comes out every six months? It seems like the health community changes its mind all the time. One minute, butter is terrible for your cardiac health and everyone recommends margarine. Within a few years, margarine is out and butter is back in. No matter what, you need to eat and drink on a daily basis, and what you eat and drink will affect your overall health.

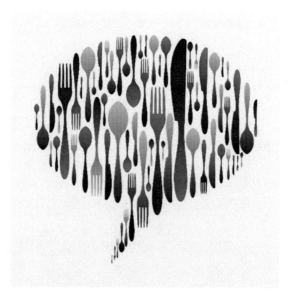

Whether you have a health condition or you're going through a time in your life where your nutrient demands are different, such as pregnancy, postpartum, training for a sporting event, or metabolic changes as you age, you need a comprehensive plan. You don't need a diet, trend, or fad. You need food recommendations that are complete and coherent and help your body to actually feel energetic and healthy.

When I first started studying nutrition in 1989, the Food Pyramid recommended 8 to 11 servings of grains every day. Then, low fat and low sodium diets were the craze. Being vegetarian became all the rage. I wanted to feel healthy, so I gave up meat and followed a low salt diet. But I felt swollen and I couldn't lose those last unwanted pounds, despite being a competitive athlete. I felt tired all the time, but I just thought it was stress from school. One day, I went to donate blood and I was declined because my blood drop floated—I was anemic. I realized then that I had a lot more to learn about nutrition.

I studied many forms of natural medicine and functional medicine. I thought I was really learning about nutrition. I did colon cleanses and detoxes, ate organic foods, took herbs and supplements, and thought I was doing everything right. I felt superior and arrogant. But looking back, even then, I still didn't have a happy digestive system. I was often bloated, I still couldn't lose those last few pounds, and I retained fluid very easily. I struggled with unhappy bowels and bad reactions to foods.

I remember having an argument with a student who was studying Oriental Medicine. She challenged me that she knew about a better system of nutrition than I did. Of course, feeling proud about all the knowledge I'd accumulated about nutrition, I rose to the challenge. When she asked me if I knew about the significance of food temperature and that different foods had an innate temperature, I had no idea what she was talking about. But I was intrigued and the conversation stayed with me.

About a year later, I found myself in Oriental Medicine School. I was finally introduced to the concept of the temperatures of foods, herbs, and spices. It was like a bomb went off in my head. The smoke cleared, and the sun shone! Knowing that subtle changes in temperature could have ripple effects in your digestion, health, and life changed my entire approach to nutrition.

I could apply these principles to everything I knew about nutrition, and it all made perfect sense. I didn't have to follow fads, diets, or the latest and greatest trends anymore. I could always sort out any information by using these principles. My digestion changed. I no longer easily reacted to foods or felt bloated, I stopped retaining fluid, and I felt better all around.

I know you want to eat healthy foods. You try to stay up-to-date with all the new diet plans, studies, and trends, but you still feel intense indecision about your food choices. You want to feel healthy and still enjoy food. You have your own food traditions, want to enjoy holidays and gatherings, and you don't want to be on a diet all the time.

So what do you do?

This book will give you a foundational perspective on time-tested Oriental Medicine and practical advice on how to eat in a way that keeps your digestion warm, your body healthy, and reduces your stress around food. I began putting these guidelines together when I started my practice and have been adding and subtracting since then as my experiences and understanding grew. In the next pages, I will break it down for you and make it easy for you to apply these principles. Throughout these chapters, I have included relevant information and wisdom I have gained from my own study of nutrition and fascination with how the body functions the best for over 25 years, which includes: over 14 years in clinical practice, clinical and epidemiological nutrition studies, biochemistry, human nutrition studies, natural medicine, functional medicine, biological terrain, Ayurvedic nutrition, naturopathic nutrition, modern research, human relationships with food, and ethnic and cultural food traditions, all interwoven with Oriental Medicine's principle of warm digestion.

What Is Warm Digestion?

First of all, having a warm digestion does not mean you have to eat a lot of spicy food! The concept of keeping a warm digestion is deeply rooted in Oriental Medicine. Think of your digestive system as a soup pot that needs to reach a certain temperature to begin to "cook" (or properly digest) the food.

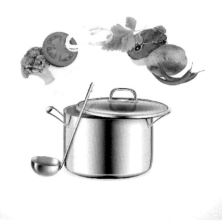

All foods, herbs, and spices are categorized and have a temperature, ranging from cold to hot. Cooking, as well as certain ways of preparing food, such as adding spices, can help change the temperature qualities of some foods. For example, iced water is cold, but you can warm water to a neutral room temperature, or you can boil it to make it hot. The more cool foods and drinks you have, the harder your digestive system must work in order to "heat" the food to properly digest.

Oriental Medicine has shown that many of our health issues dissipate when our digestion warms up. This makes you wonder why we think that eating cold salads every day is a path toward good health. What we have been taught to think is healthy may not be optimal for our digestion. Our modern grocery stores make all types of produce available year-round, but it might be better to eat certain foods in different seasons or to prepare food differently to change its overall temperature. For instance, it's actually best to eat warm, cooked foods during winter months when our system could use some warming, and wait to eat more fruits and salads in summer, when our system needs a cooling effect.

Why Don't You Want A Cool Digestion?

If your digestion is cool or cold, your ability to properly digest food is weakened. You may physically feel the effects of a cool digestion as: sluggish digestion, gas, bloating, abdominal distention, reflux, food allergies or sensitivities, irregular bowel movements, frequent illnesses and colds, or have a chronic runny nose. You may also get sick easily, be fatigued, and have difficulty gaining or losing weight. If your digestion is cool or cold for a long time, you may become prone to more severe illnesses and long-term poor health.

How To Keep Your Digestion Warm

Oriental Medicine is about seeking balance in all areas of life, including food and digestion. Having a nice mix of temperatures, flavors, and foods greatly enhances health. Preparing cool foods with spices that are categorized as warm, for instance, makes the food warmer and easier to digest. Fermenting cooler foods warms them up because the fermentation actually begins the process of digestion.

8 Ways You Can Have Warm Digestion On A Daily Basis

1. Start your day with a warm, cooked breakfast.
2. Eat cooked foods in cooler/cold weather and during season transitions.
3. Eat significant amounts of frozen foods, fruits, raw veggies, and salads only in warmer weather. Some people's digestion is naturally cool, so you may need to avoid these cold foods, no matter what the climate is.
4. Avoid eating leftovers right out of the refrigerator without warming.
5. Eat soy products in moderation, as they are inherently cold.
6. When eating dairy, choose dryer and harder cheeses (less damp and cooling), and plain or neutral flavors of yogurt. Adding cinnamon to yogurt will warm it up.
7. Have cool smoothies mostly in warmer times of year. Adding spices, such as ginger, cinnamon and nutmeg, will warm the smoothie up.

8. Rarely have drinks with ice cubes in them, unless it's summer.

Lists Of Foods From Cold To Hot

Generally

- Fruits are cooler than vegetables.
- Vegetables are cooler than grains and legumes.
- Grains, legumes, and nuts are neutral.
- Animal meats are warm.

Within each category though, there is a range of temperatures. If you're trying to warm up your digestion, you want to avoid fruits and raw vegetables, generally, but within the fruit and vegetable categories, there are some types that are cooler or warmer than others. Also, although grains, legumes, and nuts are neutral, soy is cooler than rice, and rice is cooler than oats. Let's go through the temperatures of foods within each category.

Fruits

Cold: banana, blueberry, cantaloupe, cranberry, grapefruit, mango, persimmon, rhubarb, tomato, watermelon, mulberry, plum, kiwi

Cool: apple, avocado, black current, prunes, tangerine, pear, oranges, coconut

Neutral: apricot, loquat, papaya, pomegranate, tangerine, peaches, lemon

Warm: blackberry, cherry, dates, grape, litchi, longan, quince, raspberry, strawberry, kumquat, figs

Hot: pineapple

Vegetables

Cold: asparagus, Chinese cabbage, seaweed, snow peas, water chestnuts, dandelion leaf, white mushroom

Cool: artichoke, bok choy, broccoli, cauliflower, celery, corn, cucumber, daikon radish, eggplant, mushroom, spinach, swiss chard, turnip, zucchini, alfalfa sprouts, bamboo shoots, carrot, endive, potato, romaine lettuce, tomato

Neutral: beets, carrot, cabbage, collard greens, lettuce, shitake mushroom, olive, peas, pumpkin, yam

Warm: bell peppers, chive, green bean, kale, leek, mustard greens, parsley, parsnip, squash, sweet potato, watercress, scallions, onion, fennel, oyster mushroom

Hot: garlic, green onion

Grains, Legumes, and Nuts

Cold: wheat germ

Cool: amaranth, barley, buckwheat, millet, wheat, wild rice, lima beans, mung beans, soybean

Neutral: brown rice, corn, flax, white rice, almonds, chick peas, hazelnut, peanut, pistachio, pumpkin, sunflower seeds

Warm: oats, quinoa, safflower, spelt, black bean, chestnut, pine nut, sesame seed, walnut

Animal Products

Cold: clam, crab, octopus

Cool: eggs, pork, duck

Neutral: abalone, rabbit, cheese, duck, goose, herring, mackerel, milk, oysters, salmon, sardine, shark, tuna, chicken

Warm: beef, anchovy, butter, chicken, eel, ham, lobster, mussels, shrimp, turkey, venison, fresh water fish, sheep, goat, sheep milk.

Hot: lamb, trout

Spices and Oils

Cold: salt, white pepper

Cool: marjoram, mint, peppermint, tamarind, cilantro leaf, sesame oil

Neutral: coriander, licorice, saffron, olive oil, peanut oil

Warm: anise, basil, bay leaf, carob, caraway, clove, cumin, dill seed, fennel, fenugreek, fresh ginger, nutmeg, oregano, rosemary, sage, spearmint, thyme, jasmine, coriander

Hot: black pepper, cayenne pepper, chili pepper, cinnamon, dry ginger, horseradish, wasabi, mustard, garlic

By now, you may be beginning to have a better idea about warm and cold foods and how they are affecting your digestion. This is by no means an exhaustive list! You can take these lists and experiment and even add your own foods as well. At the end of the day, you are the best judge of your body.

For a more in depth resource you can read this book: Healing with Whole Foods: Asian Traditions and Modern Nutrition by Paul Pitchford.

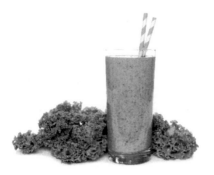

Hey, Raw Kale Trend… Meet Warm Digestion!

Recently, it has been very trendy to have raw kale salads and juice raw kale. Kale is considered a superfood and it contains a lot of beneficial nutrients. But did you know that raw kale also has substances called "goitrogens," which can disrupt the production of thyroid hormones by interfering with iodine uptake in the thyroid gland?

A simple enough remedy for this issue is cooking, which renders most goitrogens inactive. Goitrogens can also be found in other cruciferous vegetables, including cabbage, broccoli, brussel sprouts, collards, and turnips, which are also more beneficial to your health when cooked.

Damp Digestion

The term damp in Oriental Medicine can refer to external factors like a wet, rainy climate, or to internal factors like a body's tendency to retain fluids. Foods that can cause damp accumulation in the body can adversely affect digestion and overall health. Dampness accumulates in the body and produces fluids that cause imbalances in the system, especially if you have a compromised digestion and/or eat a lot of damp foods. Cold foods, dairy, sugar, processed foods, and simple carbohydrates can produce excess damp.

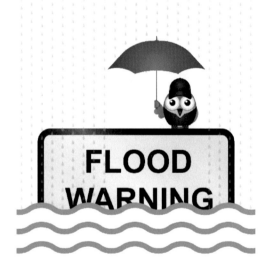

Symptoms of dampness in the body may include: easily feeling tired, heaviness in the body, increased pain in the joints, edema, as well as cysts, tumors, and imbalances to the flora in the gastrointestinal (GI) system. All of these symptoms further compound the damp conditions in the body and lead to phlegm accumulations. In Oriental Medicine, phlegm is considered to cause many different types of diseases.

But there is also such a thing as a damp-heat, which can be caused by living with stress or a long-term disease or by eating a mixture of dampness and inflammation causing foods. Some symptoms of damp-heat may be reflux, compromised lipid and cholesterol metabolism, gallstones or cholestasis, fatty liver, irregular bowels, fluctuations in appetite, and difficulty losing or gaining weight.

Here is an online pictograph, by Patricia Kowal, MAOM, L.Ac, illustrating the process of dampness and how it can affect the body:

https://magic.piktochart.com/output/3615511-dampness

Flavors Keep The Balance

The balance of flavors is what makes food taste amazing. Master chefs are brilliant at combining subtle and bold flavors. All flavors have a predominant action in Oriental Medicine. Practitioners purposely choose certain flavors and temperatures of foods to affect particular outcomes for health.

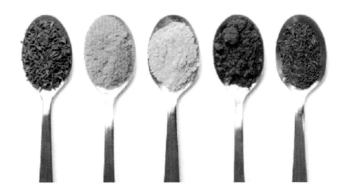

Here is a guide to help you understand the role of flavors in your daily health and digestion:

- Sour holds in and astringes.
- Bitter drains and dries.
- Sweet strengthens, moderates, and harmonizes.
- Spicy (also Acrid or Pungent) disperses and invigorates.
- Salty purges and softens.
- Bland drains damp and promotes urination.

Sour

The sour flavor has a cooling quality. As an astringent, it prevents or reverses the leakage of fluids, has a drying action, and enters the liver and gallbladder to help break down fats and proteins. Sour flavors are useful when you're experiencing symptoms such as excessive perspiration, hemorrhages, diarrhea, weak sagging tissues, hemorrhoids, and prolapses (such as a uterine prolapse). Also, when you combine meat protein with vitamin C, which is a sour flavor, you increase iron uptake in the digestion. Here are some examples:

Sour: lemon, lime, pickles, rose hip, sauerkraut

Sour and Bitter: vinegar

Sour and Spicy: leek

Sour and Sweet: apple, blackberry, cheese, grape, mango, olive, raspberry, tangerine, tomato, yogurt, sourdough bread

Bitter

Bitter is a good counterbalance when you've had too much sweet in your diet. The bitter flavor has a cooling quality, and it acts to descend, drain, and dry fluids. Bitterness helps to alleviate inflammation, damp conditions, retention of fluids, and constipation. Bitter also clears heat in various places in the body, which means it cleans arteries of cholesterol deposits and fats, clears a congested liver after eating rich foods, and counteracts dampness in gastrointestinal issues (such as candida overgrowth) and damp accumulations manifesting into excess body fat.

Because bitter reduces dampness in the body, the best season to include the bitter flavors in your food is during the fall and winter in order to protect your lungs from phlegm accumulation and to reduce your chances of getting typical winter illnesses. Here are some examples:

Bitter: mustard greens, collard greens, kale, dandelion greens, romaine lettuce, rye, oolong tea

Bitter and Spicy: citrus peel, scallion, turnip, white pepper

Bitter and Sweet: asparagus, celery, lettuce, papaya, quinoa

One more note on how to use bitter flavors in your daily routine: oolong tea is especially good for weight loss because of its bitter flavor.

Sweet

In Oriental Medicine, sweet does not refer to any type of synthetic or processed sugars—those should generally be avoided because they wreck havoc on the body's ability to maintain balance. There are two types of sweet flavors and it is very important to differentiate between them. The full sweet flavor is strengthening and generally warming, while the empty sweet flavor is cleansing and cooling.

Full sweet flavor

The full sweet flavor is found in complex carbohydrates, most dairy, and animal foods. It harmonizes other flavors (balances and moderates other flavors), has a relaxing effect, and builds tissue and fluids in the body. Full sweet also strengthens the digestion, moistens dry conditions, and calms the over-thinking and ruminating aspects of the mind. Full sweet is appropriate for every season, but most especially important during season transitions. Here are some examples:

Vegetables: beet, carrot, chard, cucumber, potato, squash, sweet potato, yam, and eggplant (caution, is a nightshade – see chapter about inflammatory foods)

Nuts and Seeds: almond, chestnut, coconut, sesame, sunflower, walnut

Empty sweet flavor

The empty sweet flavor mostly occurs in fruits and usually promotes dampness in the body, which can cause digestive issues. Moderation is the key here. As they are naturally cooling, it is better to have the empty sweet flavor in the warmer months. You can also warm them up with cooking and spices.   Here are some examples:

Fruits: apple, apricot, cherry, date, fig

A note on natural sweeteners

There are certain sweeteners that have their own useful properties. Honey has a special characteristic of drying mucous and decongesting, which is why it is used in cough medicines. Local honey also helps with seasonal allergies. Molasses, rice syrup, raw turbinado sugar (not overly processed or refined), and barley malt have similar properties to other sweeteners of harmonizing, relaxing, and building tissues.

Spicy

The spicy (also acrid or pungent) flavor is generally warming, has a dispersing quality, stimulates circulation and digestion, and breaks up mucous in the diet. The spicy flavor is useful in combating illnesses and breaks up food stagnation, especially due to cold and damp accumulations. Cooking spicy flavors tends to moderate their effects.

Warming Spicy: ginger, cinnamon, fennel, dill, anise, coriander, cumin, onion, horseradish, black pepper, sage, hot peppers, cayenne, spearmint, rosemary, scallion, garlic, cloves

Cooling Spicy: peppermint, marjoram, elder flowers, white pepper, radish

I recommend ginger and cinnamon for seasonal transitions, those who have cold or changeable digestions, and those who are inclined to mucous and damp conditions. Both of these are also great for the person who feels cold all the time.

Salty

The salty flavor is cooling, moistening, softens hard accumulations and stiffness, improves digestion, detoxifies the body, and can purge the bowels. The salty flavor is good for symptoms such as constipation, abdominal swelling, and pain. Gargling with salt dissolved in warm liquid can soothe a sore throat. Salt also detoxifies the body and strengthens mental concentration.

The alkalizing quality of salt balances acidic foods like meat, which is why it is beneficial to salt meat before cooking it. Sodium is an electrolyte in the body, which helps maintain the body's fluid balance. It is essential for water regulation, nerve transmission, and muscle contraction. It helps maintain the acid-base balance in the body along with potassium. Salt also contributes to balance electrolytes in the body.

Misconceptions About Salt

Salt has a bad reputation in our society. How often have you heard experts in the field tell you to eat a low fat, low salt diet? My question is, how many people actually feel good on that diet? I mean, truly energetic and vital?

I think of my wonderful grandmother. She grew up in the era of low fat, low salt diets when most doctors, especially cardiologists, prescribed salt restrictions all the time. In her later years, my grandmother kept getting low sodium counts in her blood work and felt weak and tired. Finally, I brought a good sea salt to her house and put it on her table. I said, "You need to salt your food!" For many years, when we spoke, she would conspiratorially tell me, "I'm still using the sea salt, but I don't tell my cardiologist!"

Whenever I gave her nutritional advice contrary to the mainstream, she always had that look in her eye. She reveled in being a little bit rogue with her nutrition after being diagnosed with Celiac Disease (gluten intolerance) in her sixties. She went on to live to the age of 96 following a gluten free diet at a time when it was not well known or understood.

Recommended Daily Allowance

The Recommended Daily Allowance (RDA) for sodium is currently no more than 2.3 g (2,300 mg) of sodium daily for healthy adults. That is equivalent to about 1 teaspoon of salt a day. According to the Institute of Medicine, the maximum daily intakes for sodium are as follows:

- Ages 1 to 3 -1,500 mg
- Ages 4 to 8 - 1,900 mg
- Ages 9 to 13 - 2,200 mg
- Ages 14 and up - 2,300 mg

All Salt Is Not Created Equal

Over more than 14 years of clinical practice and observing family, friends, and myself, I actually question the RDA. Yes, there are people who are truly salt sensitive and need to be very careful about their salt intake. But I have observed that the majority of people seem not to have enough of the right kinds of salt in their diet. I also think preparation is very important (as salting meat before cooking begins the digestive process, as well as making it less acidic). I would love to see more studies about this.

There is a belief perpetuated in the nutrition world that food either tastes good or it's good for you, but NEVER shall the two meet! I believe gourmet food recipes and trends have shown that good food can also taste amazing. If we implement the balance of flavor with good ingredients and proper preparation, not only our tongues, but also our bodies will thank us!

Synthetic Versus The Real Deal

It's extremely important to use good sea salt or salt from natural sources. Low quality salt, which usually has a synthetic sodium additive, can be harmful if overused. Regular "table" salt is composed of sodium and chloride and often has iodine added. We buy table salt because it's cheap and abundant, but it doesn't have all the trace minerals that salt from the earth or sea has.

There is a big difference in how your body utilizes synthetic salts versus real salts. I always recommend to my patients, friends, and family to use sea salts or mined salts. There are many great books and resources written on this subject, and I would highly recommend reading them. I will list some of the best starter resources for further reading at the end of this section.

At the end of the day, you need some salt in your diet—the type is up to you!

The Importance Of Electrolytes In The Body

Think of electrolytes like the spark plugs in the car of an engine. If you don't have adequate electrolyte levels, you feel lethargic and tired and your body just does not work as well as it could. The balance of the electrolytes in our bodies is essential for the normal functioning of our cells and organs. Electrolytes are present in blood, urine, in the fluid inside the body's cells, as well as in the fluid in the space surrounding the cells. Here are the seven main electrolytes:

1. Sodium
2. Calcium
3. Chloride
4. Magnesium
5. Potassium
6. Phosphate
7. Bicarbonate

The first five electrolytes in this list (sodium, calcium, chloride, magnesium and potassium) are the most common and are essential for many heart, nerve, and muscle functions.

Kitchen Remedy For Quick Electrolyte Water

For a daily electrolyte pick me up: mix 1 tablespoon of lemon juice with 1/4 teaspoon of a full sweet sweetener, like honey or raw turbinado sugar, and a pinch of salt in 6 to 8 ounces of water.

Further Reading, Links, And Resources

More about flavors and their properties:

Book: Healing with Whole Foods: Asian Traditions and Modern Nutrition by Paul Pitchford.

Pros and cons of table salt versus sea salt:

Online: http://blog.fooducate.com/2011/08/12/sea-salt-vs-table-salt-the-truth/

Pink Himalayan Salt:

Online: http://skinnywithfiber.org/8-surprising-benefits-of-pink-himalayan-salt/

Article about electrolytes and their role in the body:

Online: http://www.builtlean.com/2012/11/28/electrolytes/

We Need Fats and Oils

For decades, fats and oils were a public enemy in our culture. Many studies are finally coming out to debunk the fat myth. Moreover, we're finding out that the real reason obesity rates are rising may have less to do with fats and oils and more to do with faulty metabolisms (Hello, warm digestion!) and eating synthetic sugars, processed carbohydrates, preservatives, additives, etc. Plus, cold, damp foods and inflammatory foods, along with stressful, more sedentary lifestyles, increase the likelihood of gaining body fat.

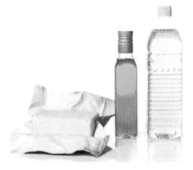

I remember a study I participated in when I was a senior in college. I interned with the AFRC Institute of Food Research in Norwich, UK. This was a heart related study where we had to drink a shake that had about a ¼ cup of safflower oil in it daily for four weeks. What stood out to me at age 21, besides the nasty taste and texture of the shake, was all of a sudden I lost weight without doing anything different than that study.

If anything, more hours spent socializing in the student union pub and eating lots of British food, one would think the opposite. But, during that study, it was very marked for me: I lost weight, my skin and hair improved, I had lots of energy and I felt really good. Previous to the study, I was always careful about anything with fat or lots of oil. To be clear, I don't recommend having a ¼ cup of safflower oil on a daily basis! But, from that study on, I realized the importance of the balance of good fats and oils in your daily diet and how they can improve your health. A lipid layer surrounds every cell in your body. Fat metabolism relies on the balance of lipids in your system. We need good fats and oils in our diets for overall health.

Now, it's trendy to have good fats in your diet and to include daily essential fatty acids, often in the form of supplements. Below is a quick guide to choosing fats, oils and supplements along with some articles and resources for further reading.

If you have a choice between anything labeled 'low fat' it is actually more healthful to eat foods unaltered with full fat intact such as: regular butter, yogurt and other dairy products. There are many full fat healthy foods such as: avocados, nuts, whole eggs, and organic meats to name a few.

Examples of Good oils

- Olive, flaxseed, sesame, grape seed, coconut, safflower.

Examples of Supplement versions

- Evening primrose oil, flaxseed, anything with Omega 3's, fish oils, essential fatty acids.

Further reading, links, and resources

The importance of oils in our diets:

Online: http://www.livestrong.com/article/267169-why-oils-are-important-in-healthy-diet/

Rethinking saturated fat:

Online:http://www.drweil.com/drw/u/QAA400919/Rethinking-Saturated-Fat.html

Online: http://time.com/3734033/whole-milk-dairy-fat/

Confessions of a Cardiologist:

Online: http://drsircus.com/medicine/confessions-of-a-cardiologist-treat-the-inflammation-not-the-cholesterol

The Vitality Of Your Food

How is it that vegetables just picked from a garden taste so different from supermarket vegetables? Wouldn't you rather eat fruit that is fresh, ripe, and in season, as opposed to fruit that was picked green and then travelled thousands of miles to the supermarket? How is it that an orange can look the same on the outside, but taste totally differently on the inside?

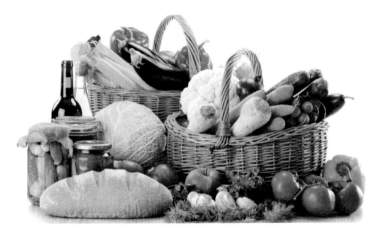

When I was a junior in college, I interned with an epidemiologist (the study of populations and their diseases) at the University of Massachusetts Medical School in Worcester. He had a lot of data from epidemiological studies from China about cancer and diets. One study stood out to me. Because of low selenium in the ground (a mineral found in the soil and essential to health in low doses) in a certain Provence in China, the overall diet was deficient in selenium. The population had a high rate of thyroid cancer. Selenium supports the thyroid and plays a role in your immunity. Because of the depleted soil, and subsequently, the food they were eating was deficient in selenium; people were getting sick at higher rates.

Now, don't run out and get a selenium supplement! I shared this study to make a point. Vitality is a concept deeply rooted in Oriental Medicine. It is the difference between feeling alive and energized, versus worn and depleted. The quality of soil and how food is grown plays an important role in food's vitality. Overworked soil, sprayed with pesticides and herbicides, can affect the nutrient quality and health of the foods grown. The vitality of farmed animals is compromised when they are raised under stressful conditions and regularly given hormones and antibiotics.

There is now a movement to buy locally grown and raised food, which indicates that our society is coming around to how the vitality of food plays a role in our overall health and enjoyment of food. If this topic intrigues you, I have included some resources to delve deeper.

Further Reading, Links, and Resources

Sustainable Agriculture, Nutrition and Flavor

"Chef's Table" (on Netflix) documentary on Dan Barber's Blue Hill at Stone Barns farm-to-table Restaurant.

Why Local and Organic foods are more vital:

Online: http://www.worldwatch.org/node/5339

Diversity matters:

Online:http://www.nytimes.com/2013/05/26/opinion/sunday/breeding-the-nutrition-out-of-our-food.html?pagewanted=all&_r=0

Anti-Inflammatory Diet: Meet Warm Digestion

If you've struggled with your digestion, have a lot of pain and inflammation or have been diagnosed with a specific disease, you may have heard of or even tried an anti-inflammatory diet.

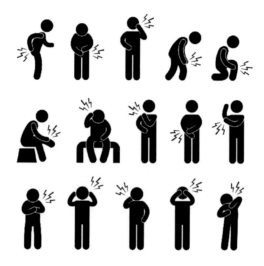

Some foods may cause physical inflammation in your digestive system, which is disruptive to a healthy digestive process. As much as keeping a warm digestion is important, some foods fall into an inflammatory category because they are hot or produce heat toxins in the body. If you are not sensitive to inflammation, you may have less trouble with these foods. But if you tend to have food sensitivities, you may have more severe reactions. Recent medical studies point to inflammation in the body as the true culprit of a lot of diseases, including arthritis and heart disease.

Many of my patients try the anti-inflammatory diet in some form or another, but find it very difficult to adhere to because it is so limiting. I find that if a person has a warm digestion, they can sometimes eat these foods without too many repercussions. Below, I list the common inflammatory food groups and then an example of how you can apply the warm digestion concept to reduce the effect of that inflammatory food in your diet. Perhaps you don't need to completely eliminate these foods; maybe warm digestion principles will be sufficient to help your body feel good while eating these foods.

Gluten

Including wheat, rye, oats, and barley, which are commonly found in breads, pasta and other products made with refined flour, is a very common allergy and inflammatory substance. Studies are still unclear as to whether it's gluten itself or some component of the grain brought out either through growth, production or preparation that causes an allergic reaction.

Warm Digestion Concept No. 1

I have found that using sprouted grains, such as bread made from sprouted wheat, greatly reduces the inflammation and sensitivity in the digestion. I also find that highly processed forms of gluten often cause more inflammation and irritation. There seems to also be a difference, based on my own and my patients' experiences, between wheat in the US and in Europe and other countries. Perhaps it goes back to how wheat is either grown or processed.

Excess Alcohol and Caffeine

Both alcohol and caffeine can affect the functioning of the liver, kidneys, and blood sugar regulation systems and have other long-term health and inflammation repercussions.

Warm Digestion Concept No. 2

Alcohol

Studies have shown the benefits of moderate use of certain types of alcohol. The health uses of alcohol go way back in time: for colds or the flu, as a painkiller, a digestive, and as an antiseptic to name a few. More recently, there are studies showing the benefits of certain components of wine for anti-aging and heart health. Red wine, in Traditional Chinese Medicine, is warming and is used in preparations of certain Chinese herb formulas to reduce pain and provide other health benefits. For postpartum patients, there is a formula where you cook the herbs in sake (rice wine) and drink this formula for the first month after childbirth. Traditional Chinese Medicine considers even water too cooling for this time of a women's life.

Formulas aside, if you were to put types of alcohol on a warm to cold spectrum, on the warm side would be red wine, whiskey, and scotch; more to the center and more neutral are white wine, rice wine (sake) and clear spirits; and toward the cool side would be beer. Any alcohol that is very sweet, like sherry or port, has a lot more sugar in it and more easily causes damp-heat and should be completely avoided if you're prone to inflammation.

Caffeine

Less processed forms of caffeine if taken in moderation can be beneficial. Generally, the decaffeination process involves chemicals that strip away the caffeine, not always effectively. Because of this, I believe it is actually better for your system to have a regular cup of coffee! Green tea, black tea and oolong tea are nice alternatives to coffee, have their own health benefits, and can help clear dampness in the body. Remember to stay hydrated with the proper balance of electrolytes as both coffee and tea are bitter and have a diuretic affect.

Soda

Soda (especially diet) and processed fruit drinks that are high in simple and refined sugars are hard on the mechanisms that regulate your blood sugar levels. High intakes of sugars, especially synthetic sugars, have been associated with inflammation and obesity.

Warm Digestion Concept No. 3

Drink more clear (less sweetened) sodas, non-diet sodas, or sodas made with real sugar. Dilute real fruit juices in water and consider it a full serving of fruit.

Meat

Pork, cold cuts, bacon, hot dogs, canned meats, sausage, and shellfish, as well as meats that are not organic or naturally raised and processed, can be high in hormones, antibiotics, and other undesired ingredients utilized during processing.

Warm Digestion Concept No. 4

Eat natural forms of meats without nitrates or additives, since they will be less reactive.

Sauces

Corn, tomato sauce, and nightshade vegetables commonly cause inflammation and allergic responses.

Warm Digestion Concept No. 5

Eat more heritage strains grown without pesticides, and eat them when they're in season.

Dairy

Eggs and dairy (all milk, cheese, butter, and yogurt.) produce dampness and phlegm in the body.

Warm Digestion Concept No. 6

Eat farm fresh eggs, harder, drier cheeses. Hormone-free milk, yogurt, and butter can be less reactive.

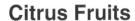

Citrus Fruits

Citrus fruits, juices, strawberries and pineapple are common allergens and/or phlegm producing. (They produce a cooling effect to the digestion). They may also adversely affect blood sugar regulation.

Warm Digestion Concept No. 7

Lemons, grapefruit and berries (blueberries, raspberries and blackberries) have a more neutral effect, help regulate blood sugar, and aid the liver and gallbladder in digestion and detoxification and reduce inflammation in the body.

Foods high in saturated fats and refined oils

Foods high in saturated fats and refined oils, such as peanuts, margarine, and shortening, may be inflammatory since processing these foods places an extra burden on the system.

Warm Digestion Concept No. 8

Less processed, good oils and fats have a true health benefit in the body's systems.

A final note on the anti-inflammatory diet

As you get to know your body and heal your digestion, you will get a better idea which inflammatory foods affect you, and to what degree. As an example, no matter how good my own digestion is, I always react to raw onions, raw bell peppers, and eggplant in any form. I also avoid synthetic sugars of any type, as much as possible.

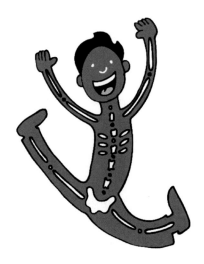

Essential Guidelines To Warm Digestion

In Oriental Medicine, warm digestion is the key to digestive health. All foods have energetic temperatures on the scale from cold to hot. Consuming a lot of cool foods will cool your digestion. To warm your digestion, you can simply change what you eat and how you prepare your food.

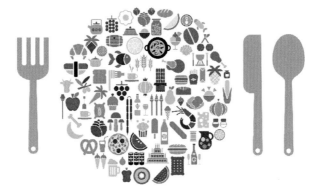

Almost any imbalance or disease begins in the digestive system. What we eat is profoundly important to our health. The guidelines in this chapter are designed as a quick-look reference for your daily nutrition.

Think of these guidelines as the center of a wheel and all other diet habits according to lifestyle, culture, and fun are the spokes. The center is always the basic diet you can come back to for good digestive health. These guidelines are appropriate for both children and adults and for most stages of your life and health.

7 Signs Of Cold Or Cool Digestion

1. Slow digestion with or without gas, bloating, abdominal distention.
2. Fatigue after eating.
3. Many food allergies, or non-specific reactions to more than a few foods.
4. Thick white tongue coating, pale tongue color, teeth marks on the side of tongue.
5. Weight gain or loss irrelevant to amount of food consumed.
6. Frequent and recurrent colds and illnesses, running nose and/or chronic congestion.
7. Irregular bowel movements.

Warm Foods And Preparations

- Eat cooked foods in cooler/cold weather.
- Generally, lean meats and cooked veggies help keep digestion warm.
- Eat significant amounts of frozen foods, fruits, raw veggies (this includes salads) only in warm/hot weather. Generally avoid if your digestion is cold.
- Substitutes for milk from warmest to coolest: oat, almond, rice, soy (coldest).

- Avoid leftovers, especially right out of the refrigerator without warming.
- Eat soy products in moderation, as they are inherently cold.
- If digestion is cool, reduce processed carbohydrates, which may congest digestion.
- Avoid eating when not hungry.

10 Daily Guidelines

1. Maintain warm digestion especially in fall, winter and season transitions.
2. Always have breakfast.
3. Always use butter, never margarine.
4. Avoid overeating or eating when not hungry.
5. Avoid foods claimed as 'low fat' or food substitutes, i.e. eggs and artificial sweeteners.
6. Choose organic foods without pesticides, hormones, antibiotics, or genetic modification.
7. Avoid refined foods and sugars.
8. Avoid too much sugar, excess caffeine, additives, preservatives, and daily intake of soda
9. Consume alcohol in moderation.
10. Eat small amounts of quality, nutrient-packed foods, rather than large quantities of low-nutrient foods.

Vegetarianism

Vegetarianism is a personal choice, often with moral implications. However, from a purely nutritional stance, in Oriental Nutrition, vegetarianism is best when practiced for limited periods and for specific issues. If you are a vegetarian, substitute meat proteins for your preferred choice of proteins when referring to this handout. Consider supplements with amino acids, such as whey or pea proteins or amino acid supplements. Common anemia's associated with a vegetarian diet can be addressed with iron, vitamin B12, and vitamin B6 supplements.

Enjoy Your Food!

A healthy digestion is a happy digestion. Slow down when you're eating and truly chew your food. Try not to multi-task when eating. Simply enjoy the moment while you're eating.

My favorite book for this is French Women Don't Get Fat: The Secret of Eating for Pleasure by Mireille Guiliano. If you want to go more into depth about the principles of Oriental Medicine and nutrition, read Healing with Whole Foods: Asian Traditions and Modern Nutrition by Paul Pitchford. The movement that's gaining global popularity is called the "Slow Food Movement," and more information is here: http://www.slowfood.com.

How To Combine Foods

The ways in which you combine your foods can aid digestion and reduce symptoms of digestive upset, such as gas, bloating, and slow digestion. In Oriental Medicine, this is called "food stagnation." If you are experiencing these symptoms, follow these guidelines for food combinations until your digestion improves.

Proteins

- Avoid combining meat proteins with dairy proteins (meat with cheese).
- Generally, protein is best combined with vegetables and grains.
- Avoid combining proteins, especially meat proteins, with fruits. Dairy proteins are less reactive with fruits. Keep in mind that dairy and fruits are both cool and both should be eaten in moderation.

Sweets

- Sugar or desserts at the end of a big meal will slow digestion.
- Eat sweets in moderation.

Life happens, so if you have mixed foods together that have caused digestive upset, usually digestive enzymes can help to relieve the food stagnation. To avoid prolonged food stagnation though, you'll want to be careful about which foods you combine.

Breakfast

- Eat warm breakfasts during the fall and winter seasons and during season transitions to protect against illness.
- Oatmeal regulates blood sugar, provides fiber, reduces phlegm and congestion, and reduces cholesterol.
- Hot grain cereals have healthful properties. Millet protects digestion, reduces nausea, and is a good wheat alternative for those with wheat sensitivities.
- Amaranth and quinoa are good sources of protein. Rice, buckwheat, and barley are especially good for weight loss.
- Have cold cereal in moderation.
- Eat sprouted grain breads because they are more easily digested and less allergenic than typical wheat bread.
- Eat yogurt sparingly, and organic is best.
- Eat meats, such as sausage and bacon, no more than two times a week.
- Eat eggs no more than two times a week.

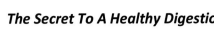
- Nut and seed butters, such as almond, tahini, cashew, and pumpkin can be good sources of protein, fats, and nutrients.

- Eat fruit in summertime or warmer climates, preferably grapefruit, apples, and berries.

- For beverages, drink green tea, oolong tea, lemon juice, or grapefruit juice. If you have coffee, make sure to counterbalance the diuretic effect it has with at least six ounces of electrolytes per cup of coffee.

- Soups may be eaten for breakfast, too.

- Consume soy products no more than two times a week. If your digestion is typically cold, avoid altogether.

- Substitutes for dairy milk are: almond milk, oat milk, or rice milk. Generally avoid soy because it is cold.

Lunch and Dinner

Lunch and Dinner should be comprised of mostly protein, vegetables, and whole grains.

Proteins

- If your digestion is weak, it is more difficult for your body to obtain protein from
grains and legumes, so lean meats are more easily digested.
- Choose lean meats of all types, preferably organic and hormone-free.
- Consume drier forms of dairy, such as hard cheeses.
- Avoid peanuts and peanut butter if prone to allergies.
- Eat tofu no more than one or two times a week because it is energetically cold.
You can sauté with ginger, garlic, and sesame oil to warm tofu up.
- Use meat substitutes sparingly, especially if sensitive to wheat.

Vegetables

- Eat any and all vegetables.
- Eat nightshades sparingly if you have internal heat, are prone to mouth sores, or
  are sensitive to inflammatory foods.
- Vegetables should, generally, be cooked, since a lot of raw veggies cool the
  digestion. The preferred cooking methods are steaming, baking, and roasting.

Grains

- White rice, especially Jasmine or Basmati is more easily digested than other
  types of rice.
- For brown rice, toasting before cooking can begin the process of breaking it
  down for more sensitive digestions. A sign that you may want to do this is a
  feeling of fullness, gas, or bloating after eating.
- Amaranth, millet, and quinoa are good sources of grains dense with nutrients.
- Choose sprouted grain breads.
- Consume lentils and corn sparingly.

Oils

- Eat more of or choose olive, flaxseed, sesame, grape seed, coconut,
  safflower
- Eat less of or avoid peanut oil, lard, and processed oil substitutes.

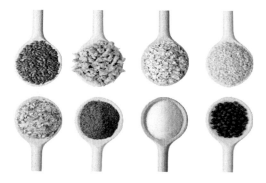

Home Remedies

I'm including a few kitchen remedies for maladies. Food is medicine, and medicine is food! Experience the effects of healthy, warm digestion in your own kitchen.

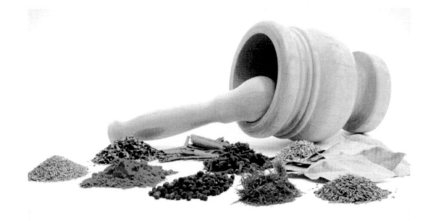

Remedies To Warm Digestion

Add fresh ginger, oregano, fennel, cardamom, cinnamon, or black pepper to the food you're cooking.

For Seasonal Colds

At the first sign of a common cold (in Chinese Medicine, we call this a "wind-invasion") drink ginger tea, 4-5 slices of ginger in boiling water, then simmer for 20 minutes, add lemon juice and honey to taste.

Slow Bowels

The liver and gallbladder can become congested which may affect the motility of the bowels. Symptoms may include: fullness below the sternum, reflux, slow digestion, phlegm, and congestion. Mix 1 teaspoon of olive oil and 1 teaspoon of lemon juice with a bit of warm water. Take first thing in morning, before food.

Quick Electrolyte Drink

Even if you drink a lot of water, you still may not have adequate amounts of electrolytes. The key to hydration and keeping up your energy and metabolism is to have a good balance of electrolytes daily. In fact, drinking too much water without balancing your electrolytes can lead to excess damp in your body causing numerous unwanted issues.

Boost electrolytes by drinking 1 tablespoon of lemon juice with 1/2 teaspoon of a sweetener (like honey or real raw sugar) and a generous pinch of sea salt in 8 ounces of water.

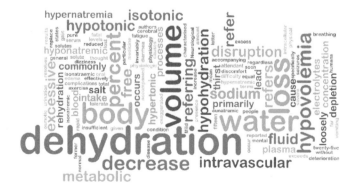

Conclusion

When I started writing this book, I asked my husband, "What does keeping a warm digestion mean to you?" He said, "Umm... drinking tepid water?" I asked my son. He said, "Umm.... not eating fruit?"

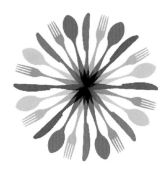

But when I observed them, the principles I have been teaching my son since birth showed through. He doesn't eat a lot of fruit, especially not out of season. He doesn't eat a lot of raw vegetables. He declines overly sweet foods, like cakes, because he says they are too sweet. When he doesn't feel well, he eats warm foods. He prefers a cooked breakfast to a cold one. Indeed, there are many more examples too numerous to mention.

My husband used to drink a pint of milk every morning. He doesn't do that anymore. He makes the most awesome chicken soup ever, which we make in huge batches, freeze, and reheat throughout the winter and during season changes. It is the most healing, warming, nourishing meal we have!

Even though he was a smoothie addict at one point, last winter he surprised me and said, "I'm not having smoothies in the morning because they are too cooling." When he does have a smoothie, he adds ginger, cinnamon, and cardamom to warm it up. He only puts ice in his drinks in summer when he is hot.

My son and husband have absorbed these principles over time. I tell you this to reinforce the idea that this e-book is NOT a diet book. I hope I have offered you a new perspective, a new way of looking at the foods you put into your body.

This book is the result of my own nutritional journey. I wanted it to be an easy to read, non-technical guide by simplifying these concepts for easy implementation. Because, just like you, I was tired of all the different types of diets that leave people not feeling very well or they are hard to implement. Just like you, I wanted to get on with life and feel better. I like to eat good food. I like to go out to my friends' homes or go to restaurants without having to worry about my diet. When my friends cook for me and ask me if I have any diet restrictions, I like to say "no" honestly.

I have an autoimmune disease that "technically" requires me to follow a specialized diet. But if I keep my core nutrition strong by keeping my digestion warm and following the general principles in this e-book, I have wiggle room to have fun and eat a variety of foods without getting off track. And if I notice my digestion becoming too cool, I can easily fix it.

Even if you just walk away implementing a few things—drink room temperature water, eat raw vegetables and fruits sparingly, eat a warm breakfast, never eat anything labeled diet or low fat, add good salt to your food, cook with good oils, eat warm proteins, and slow down to enjoy your food—then you will feel your digestion and your overall health improve. And that is something worth trying for!

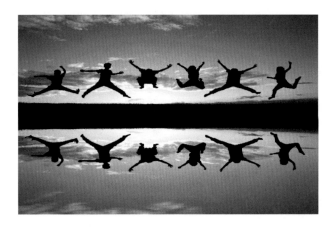

About The Author

Tansy Briggs, DOM sees patients in her practice as well as online. She regularly consults with current patients and new clients about their wellness, no matter where they live or travel.

She is passionate about educating as many people as possible about how the balance of good nutrition and keeping your digestion warm can transform your health!

Tansy Briggs, MSOM, Dipl.OM, DOM, L.OM is an Integrative Acupuncture and Oriental Medicine Practitioner. Her licenses, certificates and diplomas include: Nationally certified as a Diplomate in Oriental Medicine (Dipl.OM) by the NCCAOM (National Certification Commission for Acupuncture and 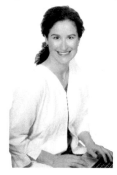 Oriental Medicine), licensed Doctor of Oriental Medicine (DOM) in New Mexico and a licensed Practitioner of Oriental Medicine (L.OM) in Pennsylvania. Tansy obtained her Master of Science in Oriental Medicine (MSOM) from Southwest Acupuncture College in 2001 in Santa Fe, NM. Prior to Acupuncture College, Tansy studied natural medicine for three years in Santa Fe via seminars and mentorships. Her bachelor's degree is from Clark University in Worcester, MA. Prior to graduation, Tansy spent her last undergraduate year abroad at the University of East Anglia, UK. You can learn more about Tansy Briggs at www.tansybriggs.com

Other Resources and References

Food lists and flavors

The food lists and flavors are adapted from the following resources:

1. Southwest Acupuncture Lectures from Doctors' Jiang Zheng and Qijian Ye for Chinese Herbs in Materia Medica, Formulas and the Classics and Chinese Nutrition.
2. My own experience from life and 14 years in clinical practice.
3. Paul Pitchford, Healing with Whole Foods, Oriental Traditions and Modern Nutrition, 1993 ISBN 1-55643-220-8.

Western Nutrition References

Cross referenced for accuracy with the following resources:

1. Whitney, Cataldo, Rolfes, Understanding Normal & Clinical Nutrition, 3rd ed. 1991 ISBN 0-314-87426-7.
2. http://www.fda.gov/Food for updated RDA.

Made in the USA
San Bernardino, CA
21 January 2016